THE NATURAL FACE LIFT

The Natural Face Lift

A Guide to Facial Exercises

Exercises to strengthen and reenergize
the face as you would your body

H. J. Maxwell

Copyright © 2005 by H. J. Maxwell.

ISBN :	Softcover	1-4134-7209-5

All rights reserved. No part of this book may be reproduced or transmitted in any form or by any means, electronic or mechanical, including photocopying, recording, or by any information storage and retrieval system, without permission in writing from the copyright owner.

This book was printed in the United States of America.

To order additional copies of this book, contact:
Xlibris Corporation
1-888-795-4274
www.Xlibris.com
Orders@Xlibris.com
26816

Introduction

Facial surgery is a temporary way of providing a more youthful appearance to the skin. Facial exercising is a more natural way of lifting the skin. The improvement can be more uniform on the entire face. The muscles are strengthened, while face surgery stretches the skin. I recommend face lifts as an optional addition along with an exercise program.

These exercises also increase blood circulation to the face, carrying oxygen and nutrients to the cells of the skin. This increases the skins ability to absorb and maintain moisture. There is an increase in the production of elastin and collagen, to substances needed for youthful looking skin.

The exercises take a few minutes per day. Five to eight minutes per day, three a days per week can provide remarkable benefits. Alternate exercises on different days, if you like. They can be done at any time of the day. Do them all at once, or individually, in between other daily activities. Do them in front of a mirror for the best results.

When you do the exercises for the first time, you will not be able to exert much force. The exercises may feel awkward. Do not be discouraged. As the muscles become stronger, you will see the improvement.

THE EXERCISES

Almost all exercises are done with the hands or fingers placed on the face. This allows for better contraction of the muscles. If done properly, it also eliminates the wrinkling and the forming of lines. Hold the hands or fingers in place firmly.

The following seven exercises can easily be done together, since the hands are kept in the same position on the face. Exercises 1c, 1d, 1e, 1f, and 1g can be done as part of exercise 9 for better results. Practice them with the hands on the outside of the face to begin with, then with the hands on the face as shown in exercise 9.

Exercise 1A

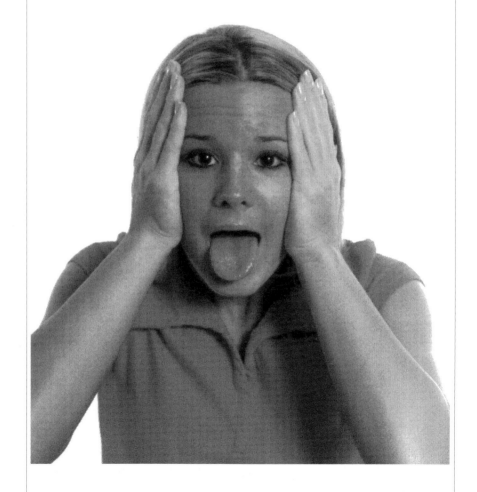

Exercise 1B

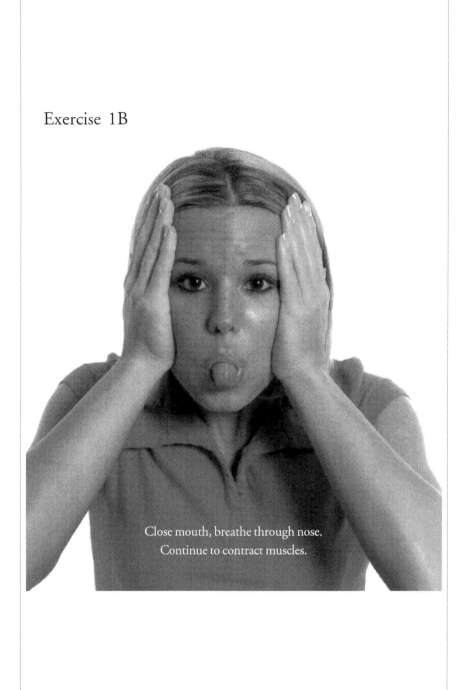

Close mouth, breathe through nose.
Continue to contract muscles.

Exercise 1C

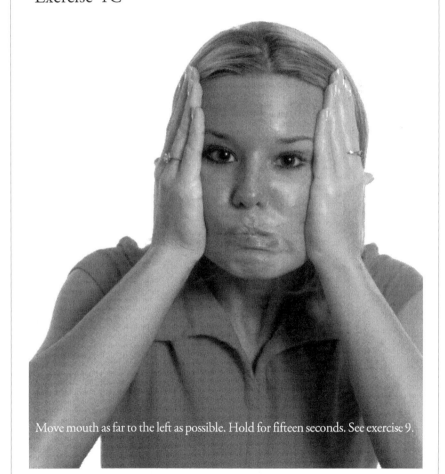

Move mouth as far to the left as possible. Hold for fifteen seconds. See exercise 9.

Exercise 1D

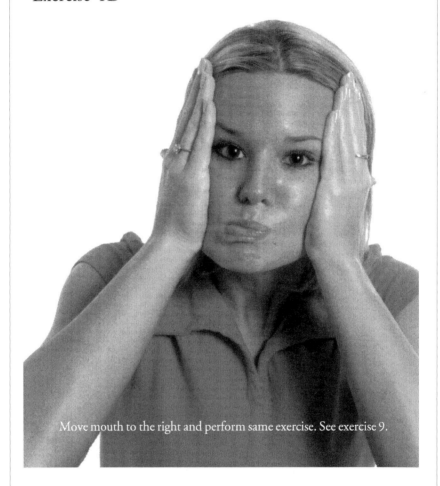

Move mouth to the right and perform same exercise. See exercise 9.

Exercise 1E

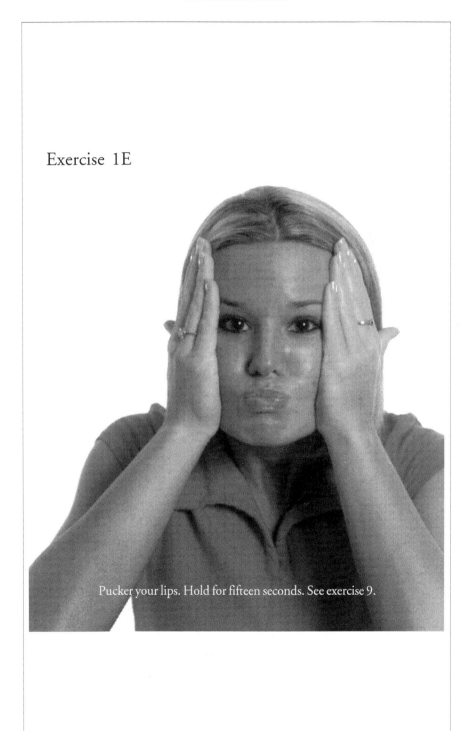

Pucker your lips. Hold for fifteen seconds. See exercise 9.

Exercise 1F

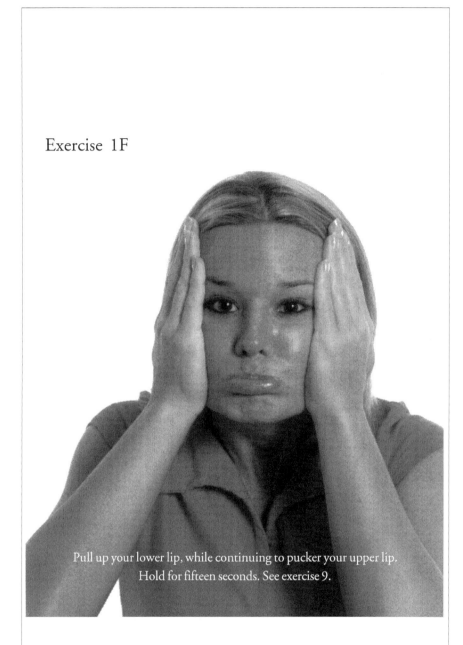

Pull up your lower lip, while continuing to pucker your upper lip.
Hold for fifteen seconds. See exercise 9.

Exercise 1G

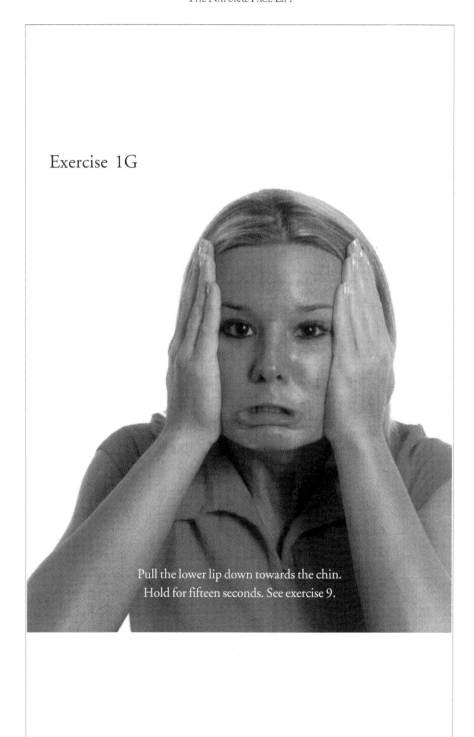

Pull the lower lip down towards the chin.
Hold for fifteen seconds. See exercise 9.

Exercise 2A

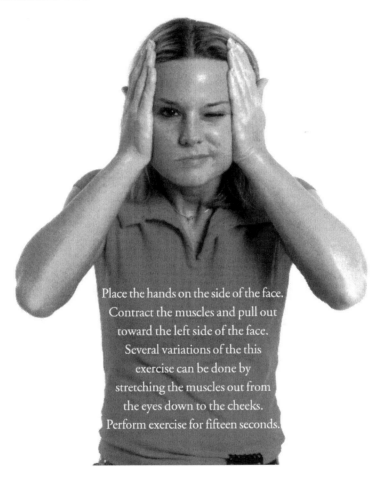

Place the hands on the side of the face. Contract the muscles and pull out toward the left side of the face. Several variations of the this exercise can be done by stretching the muscles out from the eyes down to the cheeks. Perform exercise for fifteen seconds.

Exercise 2B

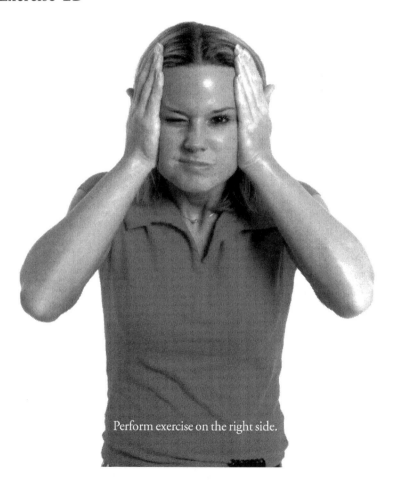

Perform exercise on the right side.

Exercise 3

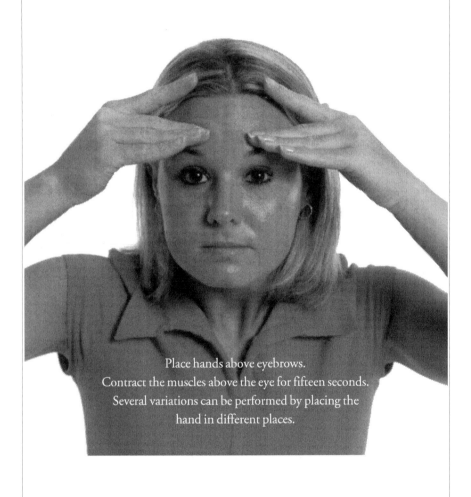

Place hands above eyebrows.
Contract the muscles above the eye for fifteen seconds.
Several variations can be performed by placing the
hand in different places.

Variation

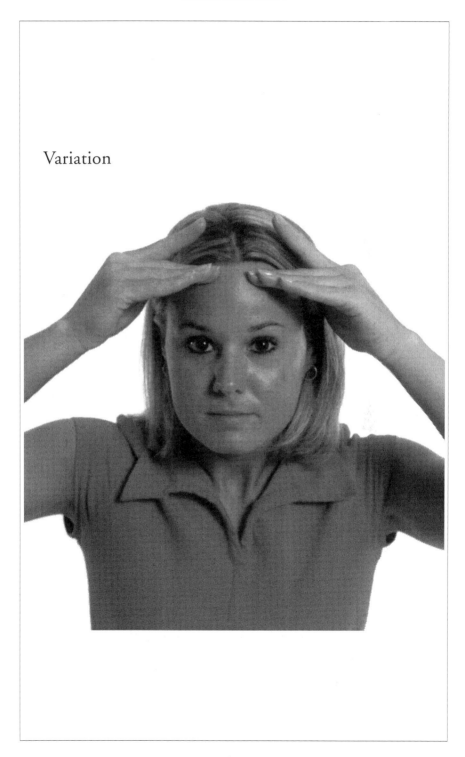

Exercise 4

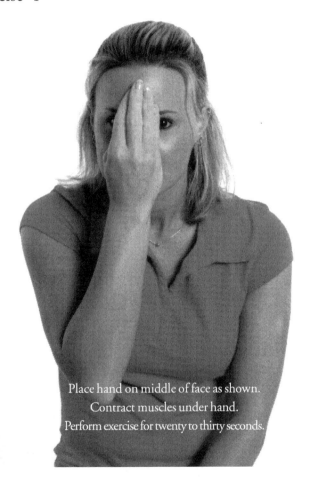

Place hand on middle of face as shown.
Contract muscles under hand.
Perform exercise for twenty to thirty seconds.

Exercise 5A

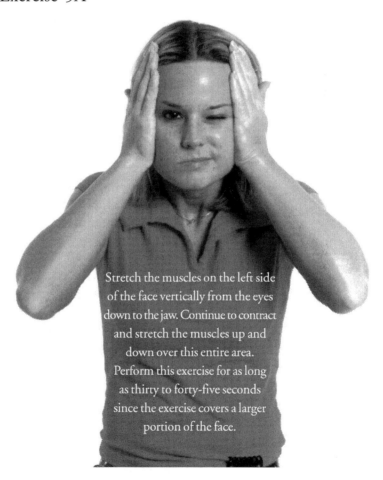

Stretch the muscles on the left side of the face vertically from the eyes down to the jaw. Continue to contract and stretch the muscles up and down over this entire area. Perform this exercise for as long as thirty to forty-five seconds since the exercise covers a larger portion of the face.

Exercise 5B

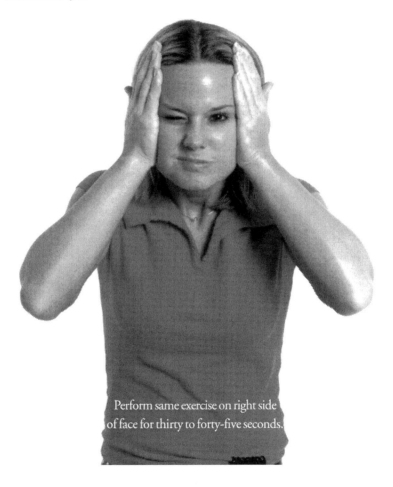

Perform same exercise on right side of face for thirty to forty-five seconds.

Exercise 6A

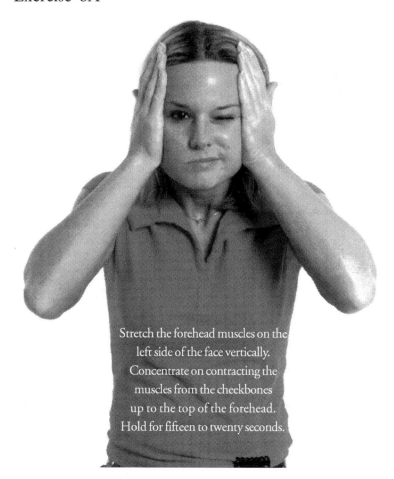

Stretch the forehead muscles on the left side of the face vertically. Concentrate on contracting the muscles from the cheekbones up to the top of the forehead. Hold for fifteen to twenty seconds.

Exercise 6B

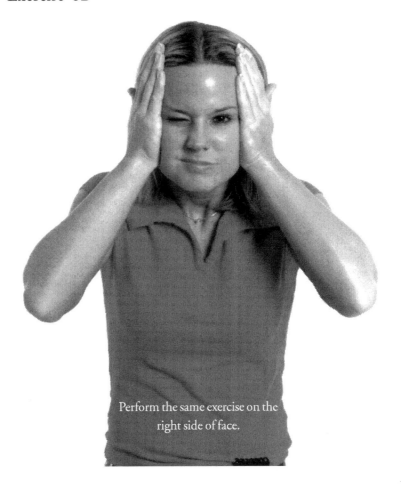

Perform the same exercise on the right side of face.

The following six exercises can easily be done together, since the hands are kept in the same position on the face.

Exercise 7A

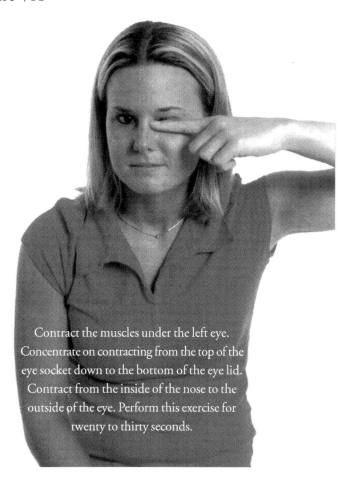

Contract the muscles under the left eye. Concentrate on contracting from the top of the eye socket down to the bottom of the eye lid. Contract from the inside of the nose to the outside of the eye. Perform this exercise for twenty to thirty seconds.

Exercise 7B

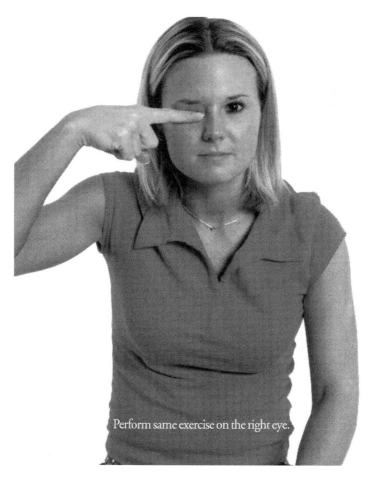

Perform same exercise on the right eye.

Exercise 7C

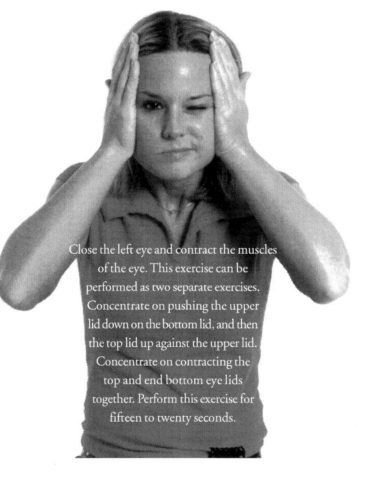

Close the left eye and contract the muscles of the eye. This exercise can be performed as two separate exercises. Concentrate on pushing the upper lid down on the bottom lid, and then the top lid up against the upper lid. Concentrate on contracting the top and end bottom eye lids together. Perform this exercise for fifteen to twenty seconds.

Exercise 7D

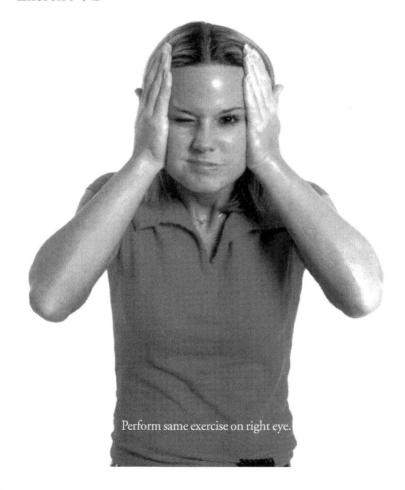

Perform same exercise on right eye.

Exercise 7E

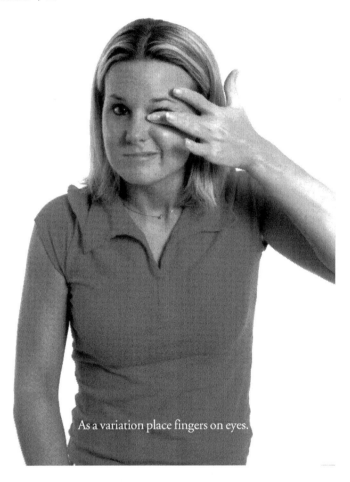

As a variation place fingers on eyes.

Exercise 7F

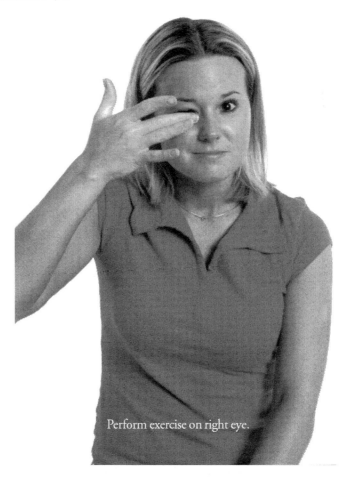

Perform exercise on right eye.

Exercise 7G

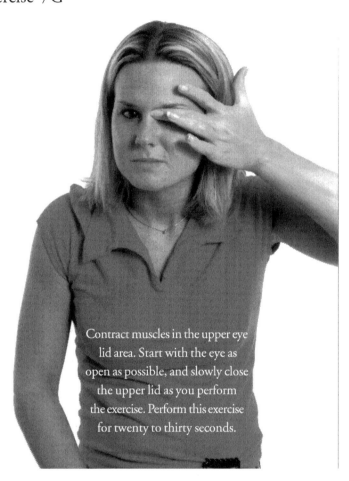

Contract muscles in the upper eye lid area. Start with the eye as open as possible, and slowly close the upper lid as you perform the exercise. Perform this exercise for twenty to thirty seconds.

Exercise 7H

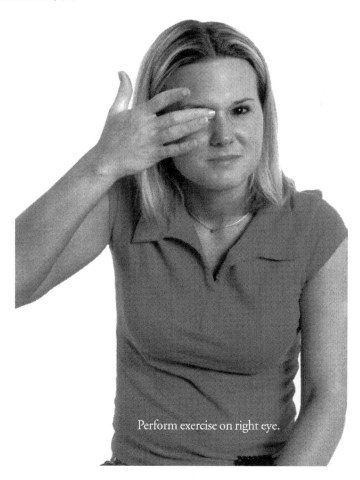

Perform exercise on right eye.

Exercise 8

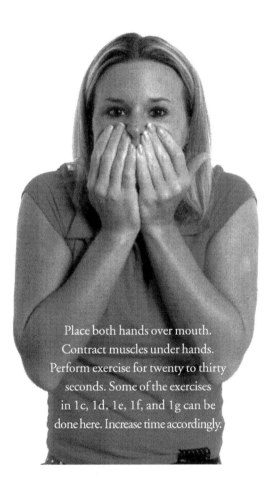

Place both hands over mouth. Contract muscles under hands. Perform exercise for twenty to thirty seconds. Some of the exercises in 1c, 1d, 1e, 1f, and 1g can be done here. Increase time accordingly.

Exercise 9

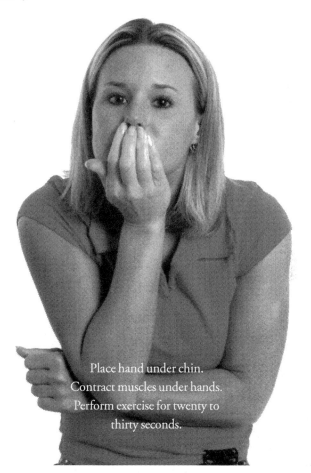

Place hand under chin.
Contract muscles under hands.
Perform exercise for twenty to
thirty seconds.

Exercise 10A

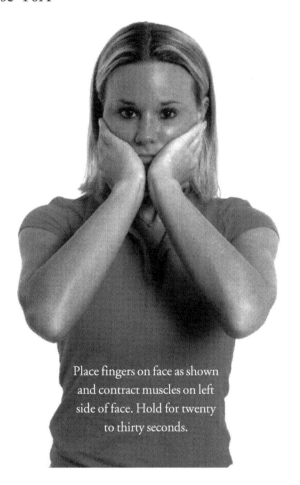

Place fingers on face as shown and contract muscles on left side of face. Hold for twenty to thirty seconds.

Exercise 10B

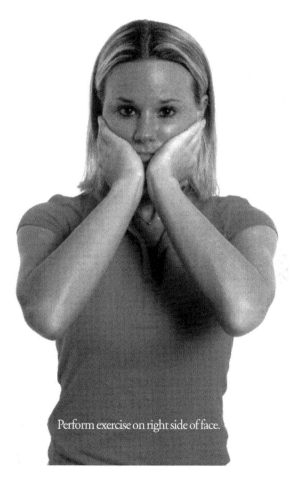

Perform exercise on right side of face.

Exercise 11

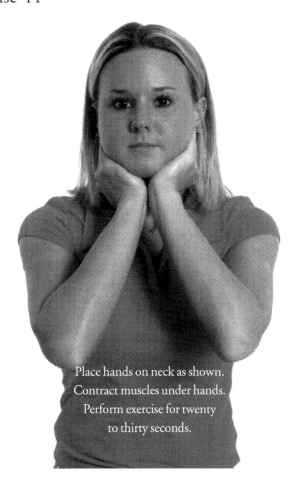

Place hands on neck as shown.
Contract muscles under hands.
Perform exercise for twenty
to thirty seconds.

Exercise 12A

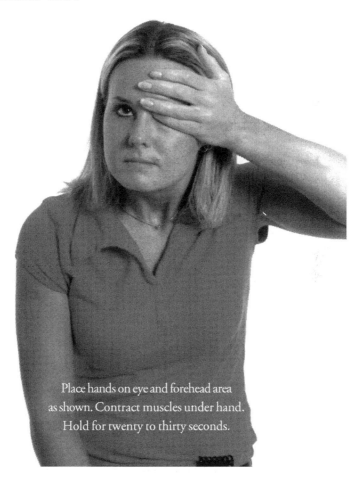

Place hands on eye and forehead area as shown. Contract muscles under hand. Hold for twenty to thirty seconds.

Exercise 12B

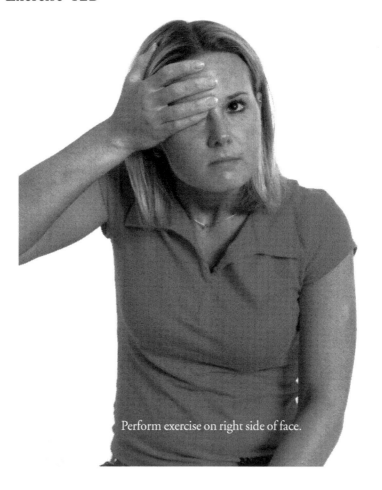

Perform exercise on right side of face.

Exercise 13A

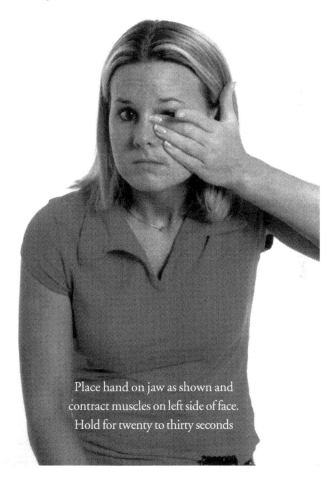

Place hand on jaw as shown and contract muscles on left side of face. Hold for twenty to thirty seconds

Exercise 13B

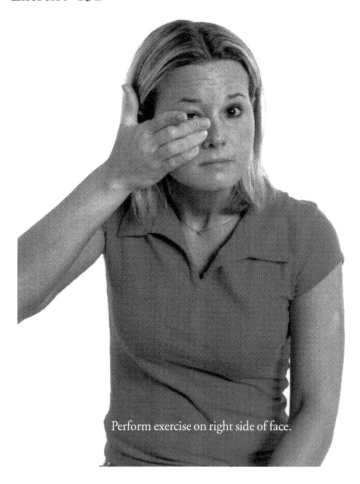

Perform exercise on right side of face.

Exercise 14A

Place hand on jaw as shown and contract muscles on left side of face. Hold for twenty to thirty seconds.

Exercise 14B

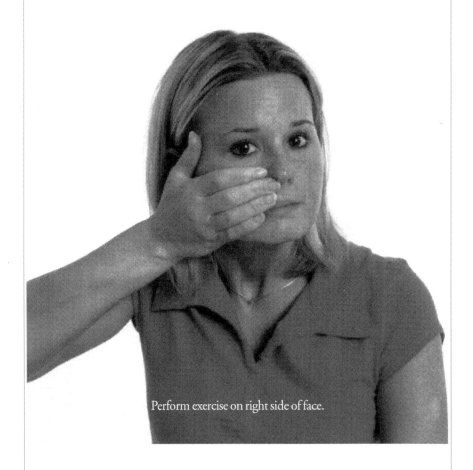

Perform exercise on right side of face.

Get your face in shape as you would your body.
See the latest in facial exercises to improve
your appearance, eyesight, and self-esteem.

Made in the USA
Lexington, KY
30 November 2010